EVERYONE wants a "miracle potion" that will melt fat away without exercise and without dieting. Most people are lazy and refuse to exercise. Some don't have the time and others can't exercise because of some debilitating illness.

And we all know that diets don't work, and we all agree that the only sure way to lose weight is to exercise and change our eating habits. But again, it's no fun to try to eat "right" all the time, to count calories, to read labels on everything we buy and to pass up the foods we truly enjoy. So, what is the answer?

CONGRATULATIONS! You have just found it! You have made one of the wisest choices in your life by buying this book because it has the answer to help you live healthier and happier in a more FAT FREE world.

LOSE FAT WHILE YOU SLEEP

No Dieting . . . No Drugs . . . No Exercise!

by

Pete Billac

Swan Publishing
Texas ❖ California ❖ New York

Author: Pete Billac
Editors: C.E. Evans, Dr. Chuck Galvin, Stuart Purcell
Cover Design: Cliff Evans and Sharon Davis
Layout Design: Sharon Davis

Other recent books by the author:

How Not To Be Lonely
How Not To Be Lonely . . . TONIGHT (for men)
New Father's Baby Guide
All About Cruises
Willie The Wisp

First printing March, 1998
Second printing April, 1998
Third printing May, 1998
Fourth printing June, 1998
Fifth printing July 1998
(Spanish version due) August 1998

Copyright @ February 1998
Swan Publishing
Library of Congress Catalog Card #98-84047
ISBN# 0-943629-33-0

LOSE FAT WHILE YOU SLEEP, is available in quantity discounts through SWAN Publishing, 126 Live Oak, Alvin, TX 77511. (281) 388-2547 or Fax (281) 585-3738 or e-mail: swanbooks@ghg.net

Printed in the United States of America.

INTRODUCTION

I am an author and publisher. I also edit and ghost write. Counting everything, I have written, edited, ghost written and/or published somewhere between 400-500 books in my life. This book is probably *the* most important one I have ever written. Let me tell you why.

First, every book that I write or publish, my main goal is to help and/or entertain—preferably both. Being an altruist by nature, I want to help others. If, in my research, I find something that I determine is of great benefit to a vast majority, I rush to tell them about it. This is such a case.

Even as I write these words, my excitement is building; I truly can't wait to finish this book and get it to the world. I think I've uncovered a true **miracle solution** to making people live a healthier, therefore happier life.

Second, the manner in which this can be done is so simple, so easy, so logical that it benefits just about everyone. It is the absolute **easiest** as well as **effortless** way to rid your body of excess fat and lose inches. Getting rid of this excess fat helps the body to heal itself.

We'll only *touch* on diets; we all know by now that DIETS DON'T WORK! This is not a diet. This is a sensible, brilliant plan that allows you to do most of what you've been doing while you feel and look better and allow your body to help in the way nature intended.

TABLE OF CONTENTS

What you are about to read in this book, in my opinion, is THE most amazing fat loss plan and product in the history of mankind. I have researched hundreds of claims on diet and weight loss plans, neither of which this is. We don't want to lose weight, we want to lose excess body FAT, therefore inches, resulting in a higher energy level and therefore becoming healthier. The body does wondrous repair on its own once we get this excess body fat out of its way.

Chapter 1

THE SECRET TO LOSING FAT

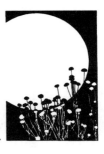

A close friend of mine, Dr. Robert M. Schwartz, wrote a book about 12 years ago titled, DIETS DON'T WORK. He followed that up about five years later with a book titled DIETS STILL DON'T WORK. Both became bestsellers. And why not? EVERYBODY wants to know how to lose weight and keep it off, but diets aren't the answer, are they?

In 1992 I received a manuscript from another friend, Lee Leva, who had been in the health club business most of his life. Lee came out with a product called FIT & SLENDER, a powdered drink, chocolate or vanilla flavor, which is superb. I still take it three of four times a week as a breakfast substitute. In it are a variety of vitamins and minerals. I mix it with water, diet cola, a little ice, vanilla yogurt and a banana. It's delicious.

For the fat burning ingredients in this drink to be the most effective, it is necessary to *exercise*. What's new, huh? We all know that exercise is essential to either become or remain strong and to tone our muscles. But what if we can't exercise? How about my friend who was stricken with polio in 1954? How can she exercise? What can she do about *burning off* fat?

And I have a host of lazy friends, don't you? Ones who just *don't believe* in exercise, or those too busy to take the time to exercise, and those who absolutely hate it. What is the answer for those who refuse to count calories and exercise? Do they just blow up bigger and bigger by the hour? Their blood pressure is soaring, as is their cholesterol, but they won't exercise or modify their eating habits until a doctor warns them that they'll die if they continue doing nothing.

About three years ago two medical doctors sent me a manuscript that I never published because it was written *by* doctors and *for* doctors, replete with medical terminology most people wouldn't understand. But, it caught my attention, and I read it carefully struggling through the "doctor" words. The words I did understand were *Behavior Modification.*

They advocated eating the *right* foods most of the time in order to lose weight and keep it off. No diet, you understand, and not doing without food, just eating in smaller portions and training yourself to be aware of and to avoid the foods with high sugar or oil content. And, of course, exercise.

They said to stay away from fried or greasy food, candy, ice cream and to count the grams of fat and count the calories in everything you eat. Who does that, huh?

It's just like using a juicer. You start with all the best intentions in the world but soon tire of a liquid diet. It's not fun feeding that noisy machine fruits and vegetables and especially cleaning it afterwards. And, you *might* be able to cultivate a taste for spinach, carrot and celery juice to where you don't gag as you drink it.

Sitting at a table for dinner with a large glass of green and yellow "stuff" is unappealing to everyone and the topic of conversation is usually centered around the juice sipper who is not invited out to eat very often.

Dining out is fun. On most first dates, the agenda is dinner and a movie, right? I cannot recall ever reading a single line in a book or watching a movie that said, "Let's diet and go to a movie." Meals are *social gatherings* of friends or family, where you eat and visit.

So, what do we have up to this point? Fit people who work out several hours a day at least three days a week who eat (or drink) foods that are no fun. We also have those who are depressed and eat and eat and eat and soon look as if they were blown up with Bavarian cream from their local donut shop. And don't forget those who have ever-expanding waistlines, hips, and thighs, that *no amount* of exercise will erase unless they adopt a regimen of eating the right foods and exercise for the rest of their lives.

Then, of course, there are those enviable ones who eat all they want and *never* gain weight. We never *really* get to like them, do we? They can just pig out at every meal and break all the culinary rules and keep their trim waistlines and enviable physique.

So, what *is* the answer? What can be done about high blood pressure, rising cholesterol level, always feeling tired, and our ever-increasing fat content? You might even *weigh* the same as you did in college, or when you were discharged from the armed services, or a year or so after you gave birth to that first or second child but that same weight has you wearing clothes that are larger than back then.

Let's face it! We are a lazy lot and why not? We are constantly enticed by televison with delicious food commercials that are downright sinful. Our highways are dotted by large signs sticking high into the sky that signal us to slow down and look at the absolutely beautiful color pictures of foods that are too appealing to pass up—and we can get this food quickly and eat it while we're driving.

STATISTICS and BODY FAT

Statistics say that we are losing the battle in the weight loss department because over ⅓ of all North Americans are overweight; 37.4 million of us are 35% or more overweight. We are, on the average, eight pounds heavier than we were 15 years ago!

It's been over 20 years since the fitness revolution began. We go to gyms, eat right, take supplements and spend over 40 billion dollars a year on weight loss and fitness, all to look and feel good. But, it isn't working. We still have a world mostly comprised of overweight people who could be healthier if they were able to get rid of that excess body fat.

Yes, look around at the people who are more than sightly to grossly overweight and if you ask, they will have a list of ailments to tell you about. Why? Because fat is unhealthy! Severely over-weight people run twice the risk of getting cancer, three times the risk of getting heart disease and up to forty times the risk of developing diabetes. And in some wild, crazy way we are losing not only our physical health but our emotional well-being. We carry around the burden of 10 or 15 extra pounds and pay the price with each bite of food. Why is this happening?

Well, it isn't entirely our fault. The *world* has changed and *we* must adapt. Our bodies were made to expend more calories throughout the day. Modern technology and our new more sedentary lifestyles have created this dilemma. We drive everywhere and rarely walk. It's gotten to the point where even walking holds many dangers.

If we want to walk around in the neighborhood, forget about a dog attacking; that's a past fear and now one of the least of our worries. We worry about getting hit by a stray bullet or some crazy person abducting us. Yes, the world has changed and we must learn to survive in it and EXCESS BODY FAT is a silent yet ever-present danger.

Because of this excess body fat we feel sluggish, we develop rheumatism-like symptoms, our cholesterol level rises, our blood pressure goes up, and our body doesn't have a chance to repair itself. So what do most of us do? We diet. Let's talk about diets for a moment.

DIETS

I am not going to attempt to "beat up" on all the diets, diet books, diet tapes, diet videos or diet doctors. I'm just going to appeal to your experience and logic.

With most diets, you are losing weight either by starvation or deprivation. Starvation means just eating less calories. Deprivation means choosing only specific food groups and eliminating others to change the way your body assimilates fat. In theory it works, but in the final outcome, the body gets its revenge.

Unless you adopt this diet forever, it just doesn't do you any good. Your body has become *accustomed* to what you have been eating for years and if you change it, the body balks. *Losing* weight is hardly the problem; *keeping it off IS!*

LOW CALORIE DIET

Just for the fun of it, let's explore a low-calorie diet. This is a diet specifically of starvation. Since you are changing the amount of available energy in terms of the intake of calories, your body immediately begins to look for other energy sources and since none are available, the body begins to convert the available carbohydrates that you have into energy instead of making protein like it's supposed to.

Having used up a lot of the body's carbohydrates, your body now begins to reduce the protein *synthesis* (the process of making a compound by joining together elements, simpler compounds or radicals) in order to conserve energy. The result is a LOSS OF BODY MASS! You are tickled pink. Who said a low-calorie diet doesn't work? But, this loss of weight is the loss of muscle, tendon and ligament as well as fat.

Next, your body begins to send you danger signals like fatigue, irritability, and loss of concentration. And then your friends (the ones who will tell you the truth) will say, "Gosh! You've lost weight—but you *look* terrible!" You know they are correct because you also *feel* terrible!

The next thing you do is abandon this low-calorie diet just to feel better. That's when your body shouts to you again. "It's about time," it says. "You lost 30% of our muscle mass and 50% of our reserves of energy."

So you eat more calories to rebuild what you lost but the *body automatically adds* a few extra pounds of reserve energy to prepare for another of your unwise decisions to diet.

LOW FAT DIET

You now want to try a diet that is low in fat. A sudden loss of fat means your dependency on carbohydrates and protein has to go up! You see, fat, carbohydrates and protein are staples of our existence, therefore a low-fat diet is one of deprivation!

Usable calories for energy comes from sugars that are stored in fat, so if fat is taken away, the body turns to the carbohydrates for its energy. Here is where you lose again. Let me explain.

When you restrict fat, your body begins to consume carbohydrates. By decreasing the carbohydrates, the body is forced to create more fat, which causes the body to increase fat accumulations. So in essence, a low-fat diet *makes* you fat!

LOW CARBOHYDRATE DIET

A low carbohydrate diet forces the body, in most cases, to conserve the fat energy it already has. Otherwise, it would have to begin using protein to make energy which is very inefficient for the body. Once the carbohydrates are at minimal levels, the body starts using the fat. Then, eventually, it turns to the protein to retain the proper energy forces it needs, and you actually begin to **lose weight!** Good news, huh? Not quite.

Because, the loss of protein also **reduces the muscle mass** and the ability to rebuild and repair itself. So, what you're losing is muscle as well as fat and that is *not* a good idea. Let's try something else.

HIGH PROTEIN DIET

This is the **LEAST DESIRABLE** diet you can possibly go on! The theory is that it takes more body caloric energy to digest protein than carbohydrates or fat. Therefore, you lose weight by burning more calories in the process of protein synthesis.

But, unless you have a rare body type that can deal with this extra protein metabolism, by increasing protein synthesis you produce an excess of *toxins* which can't get from the kidneys fast enough, and the result could be kidney stones, bad breath or *toxemia.* (Toxemia is a condition of blood poisoning, especially poisoning caused by bacteria toxins transported through the bloodstream from a focus of infection.)

In plain words, ALL DIETS ARE HARMFUL TO THE AVERAGE BODY if they starve or deprive the body of what's natural to it. In the last few decades, all sorts of diets have come on the market and they all claim to be "the" answer. If so, where are they now and why are we always trying new ones?

However, modern technology, along with Mother Nature, has given us the **solution** we have all been awaiting. It is a breakthrough in the weight/fat loss field. Let's talk about it because it might just change (or save) your life!

★★★★★★★★★★★★★

On the following page is a *before and after* photo of Dr. Mark Evans. His testimonial is not as profound as thousands of others I have in my files, but I feel most can identify with Dr. Evans, those who need to lose just "some" weight.

"In 12 weeks I lost only 14 pounds, but **24 inches** overall; 4 from my waist alone. I had tried various other weight-loss products and plans and NONE worked! I always gained the weight back.

"As a psychologist I've dealt with patients with weight challenges for years. This system has proven to be *the* effective tool to provide physical/mental health intervention. This system works on nearly everyone when it is followed correctly."

I questioned Mark on his photos. "Only 14 pounds Mark? It looks like about 40 pounds." This is a perfect example where lean muscle replaced FAT. Look at the SIZE difference in his chest and stomach.

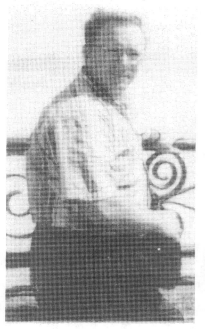

Before

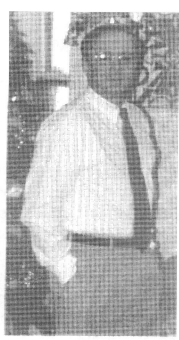

After

Chapter 2

MIRACLE SOLUTION

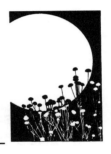

It was in the early 1980's, that Michel Grisé, a brilliant Canadian formulator, worked in the Veterinary Department of ABBOTT Laboratories in Montreal, Quebec, Canada. A veterinarian friend of his who worked for the Department of Agriculture of Canada asked him to formulate a food supplement to help reduce body fat in chickens!

Perhaps you've seen these egg-laying factories where hens are squeezed tightly in cages where they are fed and watered and remain in confinement until they can no longer produce eggs. These chickens couldn't exercise and they got fat and developed what is called *Fatty Liver Syndrome.* Their egg production lessened dramatically long before their egg-laying days were scheduled to be over.

It was impossible (certainly impractical) for these chickens to get exercise. There had to be a way to take the fat off so they would begin laying their normal supply of eggs without letting them out of these cages.

So they formulated a dry solution of additives and mixed them in with the chicken feed. Within five days, the body fat of the chickens was *reduced* and egg production went up! The Canadian beef, poultry, and dairy industries also experienced the same results with this formula. That's where the really *great* news begins.

Michel discovered that he was 30 pounds overweight and went to his doctor who put him on a 1,200 calorie a day diet. It didn't work. "This, of course, was an impossible task," Michel smiled. "I was traveling at least three days a week and had to eat hotel food. How can you eat but 1,200 calories in any one day? I was losing nothing." The doctor then suggested an 800 calorie a day diet.

"I decided that, due to the dramatic success of the product I used on the poultry, I would modify the formula by converting it from a powder to a liquid and test it on myself.

"By simply taking a tablespoonful of this new solution with a glass of water on an empty stomach each night just prior to going to sleep, I lost fat, weight, and gained more muscle tone. I lost 20 pounds in five weeks and two inches disappeared from my waist. I gained two inches across my shoulders. I did not exercise nor did I modify my eating habits!"

Michel then decided to offer the product to others. The results were spectacular. "This began in 1983. In the few years that followed," Michel added, "thousands of people lost fat and inches while preserving and building lean muscle mass. And up to this time, *tens of thousands* have experienced the same results." He named his discovery CALORAD.

With the help of an obesity specialist in Montreal, the first *clinical study* was conducted that consisted of testing 354 patients for 90 days. Neither their diet nor exercise patterns were changed.

The success rate of FAT LOSS was an outstanding 86%

HERE ARE THE ACTUAL FINDINGS

152 of the 354 tested had results in 1-30 days. (42%)
76 of the 354 tested had results in 30-60 days. (21½%)
77 of the 354 tested had results in 60-90 days. (22½%)
49 had little or no visible fat loss. (14%)

(There were benefits **other** than fat loss from this test. The testimonials is Chapter 3 will list some of them.)

HERE ARE THE SIMPLE INSTRUCTIONS

✔Take one tablespoon of CALORAD with eight fluid ounces of water on an EMPTY stomach just prior to sleep.

✔Your LAST meal should be at least three hours before taking Calorad.

✔No snacks or drinks other than water during those three hours prior to closing your eyes and going to sleep, not watching TV or reading, etc.

Does this sound too difficult for you? Remember, **NO DIETING and NO EXERCISE**.

Rena Davis, renowned clinical nutritionist, who in 1984 monitored 300 patients (ages 17 to 77) were given Calorad in her St. Helens, Oregon Clinic for a period of one year. These were **her** findings:

⏩ The AVERAGE weight loss for one year was **9 pounds of FAT** and **3.75 inch loss per month.**

⏩ Patients were not placed on a calorie restrictive

diet. (In other words, they ate what they had been eating prior to the study.)

▶▶ HYDROSTATIC (water) weighing was used to determine BODY FAT loss and LEAN MUSCLE MASS development.

▶▶ Patients were NOT required to exercise.

▶▶ 36% of the group gained LEAN muscle mass.

▶▶ Calorad was proven to be reliable and safe.

▶▶ The only side effects were POSITIVE ones.

Rena Davis took Calorad herself after having a child and lost 38 pounds. She reports her findings:

"These results were established over *13 years ago!* Since then, tens of thousands of people have achieved dramatic fitness and wellness results by using Calorad. Does this sound too good to be true? That's what I said before I reviewed the information and received the results for myself! The results have been phenomenal! It's too good not to share with you!"

THE PLAN

Take a (measuring) tablespoon of Calorad as is prescribed, and live your normal life. **That's it!** Do you understand? **THAT IS IT!** Calorad works while you sleep. Calorad works with or without the human will! Could it be any simpler? When you lose fat, you look great, as well as having more energy and stamina.

And, since fat is 2½ times as bulky as lean muscle mass, you lose **INCHES!** I know, this is just too easy, isn't it? And it is! I didn't believe it when I was first introduced to it but—**IT WORKS!**

UNDERSTANDING CALORAD

Many people will try *anything* to lose weight. So why not TRY Calorad? Calorad is phenomenal and will bring a healthier life to just about everyone who takes it. But Calorad can't do it all alone. It is **not** a license to eat an entire cheese cake or to go to one of those *all-you-can-eat* places until you feel you've gotten your moneys worth. It is merely a *better way of metabolizing your fat* the way nature intended.

For example, as children we produce large amounts of growth hormone which causes the body to convert and metabolize stored energy and produce muscle, tendon, and ligaments for growth.

As adults, growth hormone production slows, leaving us the option of using collagen instead to complete the same task. And, not *all* collagen products do the same job as Calorad does! Calorad is a formula *with* collagen as a primary ingredient. Let's now understand more about . . .

COLLAGEN

Collagen comes from animal products, usually beef connective tissues. Collagen is essential in the formation of strong muscle, tendon, ligaments, skin, nails, and hair. The **lack of collagen** causes the skin to hang, wrinkles to form, nails to break. A general body weakness develops simply because the body can't repair itself properly.

So, collagen is used in the protein synthesis to combine with the energy source—fat—to produce the necessary proteins that the body needs to repair these muscles, ligaments, and tendon. Now that we have collagen, let's find out how the body does the work.

Almost all body repair takes place during the *Alpha* phase of the brain's sleep cycle—the first several hours of sleep. The process involves the body shifting gears from the awakened *Beta* cycle of brain behavior that takes place during the day to a restful, rebuilding, rejuvenation behavior during sleep.

During this period of sleep, the body uses the available collagen and other vital nutrients and coverts them into new body materials. This process takes an enormous amount of caloric energy to complete and that's why one may wake up a few pounds lighter. What happens is an individual will *burn off* some calories by metabolism to make new body repairs during sleep. Therefore if one is deficient in collagen, you can't burn off the fat or repair the body very effectively.

Now, as wondrous as Calorad is, it is not to be used as a meal replacement; you need to eat three regular meals per day with the normal intake of 2,000 to 2,500 calories.

If you already exercise, there is no need to increase your exercise program since you'll be burning more calories by metabolism. But if you begin to exercise, or increase your exercise, *of course* it will have a faster effect on your body as any food would.

To assist your body in the removal of toxins and to work more efficiently, you should drink 8 to

10 glasses of plain water per day. Actually, you should be drinking this much water anyway regardless of the program. Water is the universal cleanser.

About a dozen years ago, a friend discouraged me from drinking iced tea with my meals because of the tannic acid in it; that it might give me gall stones or kidney stones. I didn't know if it was right or wrong but I listened; it's cheaper anyway. I know for certain that it changes—maybe improves—the taste of water.

One ounce of lemon juice (about the contents of one medium-sized squeezed lemon) supplies the body with 13 milligrams of vitamin C, about 22% of the RDA for adults.

Lemon in water is healthy; lemon is a neutralizer. It's involved in the pH balance in your body. So, skip the iced tea, the coffee, the coke, and drink water with some lemon in it.

Just before falling asleep, mix a **measuring tablespoon** of Calorad in an 8 oz glass of water and drink it. Remember that you want to catch the **beginning** of the Alpha cycle of your sleep. There's no need to put additional Calorad in your water. One measuring tablespoon is sufficient.

And, have an *empty stomach*. **Stop** all eating and drinking (other than water) at least three hours

BEFORE you take your Calorad in that glass of water (four hours if your digestive process is slow), after a full meal. If you had a salad or a light snack—two hours.

Finally, the entire program is based on a **3-month** plan. Everyone is different and personal results will vary. Besides, nature works best over time. Since it took many of you years to gain this body fat, it's ludicrous to expect it to just vanish overnight. We can't rush Mother Nature.

Remember, you are helping what the body does **naturally**. You are changing *metabolic function*, not going on a diet. DIETS DON'T WORK!

WHAT IS CALORAD?

Calorad is a *food* which has 14 calories; four grams of protein, zero grams of fat, and one gram of carbohydrate per one tablespoon serving. The collagen in Calorad is extracted from certified healthy bovine collagen. Each batch of collagen is inspected for purity by the Canadian government and additionally by private laboratory analysis.

Unlike any other collagen product on the market today, Calorad is the result of a **very specific extraction process** by Michel Grisé, the Canadian who created Calorad. Michel discovered a specific amino acid combination which is the key to Calorad's high success rate. Calorad does, in fact, have a certain *magic* to its formulation that many health practitioners describe as, "The most amazing nutritional supplement they have ever come across."

Calorad is being used by many consumers as a weight or inch-loss product. For those who carry around excess fat, it supports the building of **lean muscle tissue** which assists the body in burning sugar and fats more efficiently. Calorad does not stimulate, starve, or *trick* the body into weight loss. It does not require calorie counting, restricted diet, or exercise. This breakthrough formula feeds the body with a collagen-protein supplement resulting in the body shedding excess fat and toxins—**naturally!** Calorad supports lean muscle mass and facilitates FAT loss, consequently causing people to lose inches! Most lose a pant or dress size before they shed a single pound. Some will lose both weight and inches the first week, whereas others not until the end of the third month—and for some never.

Calorad, as I have previously stated, has a proven success rate. The formulation is designed to provide a highly bio-available fuel that each body utilizes according to its individual needs.

That's why not **all** Calorad users will see immediate results. The body may be using the collagen-derived amino acid components of Calorad to repair connective tissue damage of collagen disorders rather than using the product to facilitate an increased metabolism of fat or increased muscle building.

However, Calorad has demonstrated to have produced beneficial results on just about eight out of 10 of those who use it for 90 days. Test it for a month if you choose, but **three months** is the true test.

For those of you who are underweight or in good physical condition, Calorad assists the body in toning and can be used for increasing your energy level and stamina. Body builders and athletes are getting great results using Calorad before workouts. Consumers with a wide spectrum of health challenges are finding that this wellness formula is feeding the body with the perfect food for their needs.

Because Calorad is safe and effective, and **does not** require dangerous caloric restrictions, many chiropractic, naturopathic, and medical doctors are utilizing Calorad personally and professionally as a part of their total health program.

SIDE EFFECTS OF CALORAD

One of the **amazing** side effects we've found is *weight loss*. Calorad's primary effect is to stimulate the body to rebuild muscle, tendon, and ligaments. And since the process does not interfere with any other bodily function, it has no effect on medications. It can have a **positive** effect on cholesterol, and on diabetics.

Pregnant or lactating women should not take Calorad. Nor should prepubescent children, unless prescribed by a doctor.

In taking Calorad, at first you might experience a slight weight GAIN! Why? Because muscle weighs more than fat and the initial conversion of fat to lean muscle mass can result in momentary weight gain. But don't worry, it quickly reverses and goes in the other direction.

If you don't seem to be losing weight after the first 30 days, remember, the object is to *convert* fat by metabolism and protein synthesis into lean muscle and your body might choose to change its appearance first. That's why I recommend that you judge Calorad with a **tape measure**—by the way your clothes are now fitting—not a scale. The weight that begins to drop off will take place on its own time, when it's good and ready,

and not before. It's really INCH LOSS and FEEL-
ING BETTER that is advocated. That's why a full
3-month program is recommended.

Weight loss can sometimes be quite dra-
matic and very sudden. Still, don't worry. Your
body is doing what is perfectly natural for itself.
Unlike crash diets, losing fat to metabolism simply
uses the fat and doesn't hurt the body.

THOSE WHO CAN NEVER LOSE WEIGHT

There are people who, no matter what they
do, will NEVER lose weight. The reason(s) are. . .

✔You may have a malfunctioning thyroid
gland. The thyroid gland controls ALL BODY
METABOLISM. For those who suspect a thyroid
problem, it's wise to have it checked and corrected
by a physician *before* you begin any weight man-
agement program. When thyroid medication gets
your condition under control, *then* resume Calorad.

✔Due to the extensive use of antibiotics and
drugs in this country, we have changed the natural
body chemistry and flora of our intestinal tract.
Therefore, all the good and necessary body bacte-
ria and microbes have been reduced, in some

cases, destroyed all together. This has led to a silent infestation of YEAST, better known as *Candida Albicans*.

Candida is totally devastating to the body and only occurs when the body's good bacteria is no longer present to keep the yeast in check. Candida is most famous for *vaginal yeast infections* or skin rashes, but the hidden effects are far more devastating.

Yeast coats the stomach and the intestines and other organs with a thick layer of mucus. This mucus coats *bacilli*, or the outer linings of the organs, and effectively stops the transfer of nutrients into and out of the body. Therefore, you take *in* food but *absorb* very little of it. The result is, you always *feel* hungry and, eventually, overeat causing further accumulations of excess fat.

Candida is a nightmare to get rid of. There is no medication that effectively eradicates Candida; it only controls it. If you have yeast in your system, it becomes very difficult to achieve weight management. This means you'll not only never lose weight, but probably gain a few pounds per year no matter what you do.

But, there is an answer to **that** problem also. It is called . . .

AGRISEPT-L

Along with Calorad, Michel Grisé went one step farther and formulated Agrisept-L, a synergistic blend of natural **anti-viral, anti-bacterial, and antifungal properties** found in citrus. This biological formula was developed from the seeds of grapefruit, lemons and tangerines and helps to eliminate all non-wanted bacteria and microbes in the body.

It is nontoxic and has demonstrated in live blood cell testing to be helpful against the Candida Albicans outgrowth as a preventive treatment that subdues the fungus and assists the body on a weight loss program.

Agrisept-L addresses the problem of **CANDIDA**, as well as other inhibitors to weight loss including **HERPES, INFLUENZA, STREPTOCOCCUS, FUNGUS, PARASITES, STAPHYLOCOCCUS, SALMONELLA, ECOLI**, and **TOURISTA!** This natural product has NO harmful effects.

In an interview with Monsieur Grisé, I recall him mentioning that in the experimental stages of Agrisept-L, he put three liters (less than one gallon) of Agrisept-L into a **MILLION** gallons of *heavily polluted* water. "Within five hours, you could drink the water," he smiled.

YEAST TEST

The *amount* of yeast you have in your system will determine how quickly it can be removed. A quick way to determine how much yeast you have is to conduct a simple test.

Yeast can be detected in saliva. Put a glass of water on your night stand before retiring. First thing in the morning immediately upon arising (even before clearing your throat or brushing your teeth) is to gather some saliva in your mouth and *spit* it into the glass. Within minutes, if there is any yeast in your system, the saliva will immediately clump together and begin to "leak" down into the glass of water in tentacle-like fashion. It resembles a jellyfish if you've seen them under water.

If the saliva sinks down to the bottom of the glass quickly, you should consult a Health Professional to begin a cleansing program.

To **correct** Candida you could try 5 to 10 drops of AGRISEPT-L in juice or water twice a day just before meals until all signs of yeast are gone. Agrisept-L is somewhat bitter but in orange juice or apple juice, it is almost tasteless. I say stir it as you drink because it tends to settle on the bottom and that taste IS not pleasant.

Because you have signs of a yeast problem,

you may still take Calorad. It has been proven that you **can** take Agrisept-L while you are taking Calorad, but take the Agrisept-L with meals and make certain of the three hours with an empty stomach before you take Calorad.

As a **preventive** measure, add a few drops of Agrisept-L into the juice of your choice before at least just one meal daily. Agrisept-L has been laboratory tested with astounding results.

If there is NO YEAST in your system, the saliva will simply disburse on the top and not sink. Then, your Calorad plan has a better chance of working.

CALORAD ALSO HELPS BUILD MUSCLE

Athletes who want to BUILD their bodies for strength without using steroids or other harmful dietary aids can do it with Calorad. The only **change** you have to make in this program is to take your Calorad IN THE MORNING, not at night. And take it one-half-hour before **beginning** your workout.

This way, you will still lose fat weight because you are taking it in the *Beta* phase of your brain function—the daytime but **more** fat LOSS only occurs in your sleep during your *Alpha* cycle of your brain function. Even then, you'll still enhance your muscle, tendon, and ligaments.

OTHER POSSIBLE EFFECTS

Again, there are at least 500,000 Calorad users; perhaps as many as 1,000,000. The problems I ran across with friends who first began taking Calorad were simple ones.

A mother of 60 and her two sons, ages 38 and 42, complained that the first few nights on Calorad they each experienced slight stomach cramps. It was recommended that they take **half** the amount (one-half tablespoonful) in their eight ounces of water until the slight discomfort ceased.

It was explained to me by a physician that some people have this temporary discomfort because the body is flushing out toxins. The first night on a half dose, the discomfort ceased. Three more nights they tried half the usual dosage. By the sixth night on to several weeks they went back to the full tablespoonful of Calorad without any problems. Soon, they lost inches and began to feel more strength and energy.

Another lady, in her early 60's, called about cramps in her lower abdomen the first two nights she was on Calorad. Again, the half dosage was recommended. She still had slight cramps, but cut the dosage a bit more and in three days was back on the full program. I called her the following week and she feels an increase in energy and a lesser desire for food.

Several of my male friends, ages 35 to 55, reported an increase in urination during the first few nights of taking Calorad. The same thing happened to me. Within a few days for all of us, this stopped and we all began sleeping more soundly. The reason for this was a sudden increase in protein into our bodies and we were (again) flushing out unwanted toxins.

Again, Calorad is SAFE! It is an ALL NATURAL FOOD SUPPLEMENT that can only help the body help itself!

In this next segment are testimonials of those who used Calorad from one to three months and longer. Their reports were edited only slightly to avoid duplication. If you read through them, chances are you'll find one that interest you particularly.

Chapter 3

LIVING PROOF

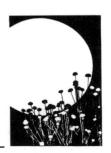

I know there are many questions you'd like to ask about Calorad that might pertain to your personal situation. These are in the chapter *following* this one. I wanted to put these testimonials here to really excite you.

As you know, I am not a medical doctor nor a nutritionist and, to be perfectly honest, I didn't believe it either. But it *sounded* so good, and it was too simple and too inexpensive **not** to try. Here is what happened to me and some friends of mine who began taking Calorad only six weeks ago.

My Experience:

For me, I slept soundly the first night I took Calorad for the first time in well over a year, and I continue to sleep soundly. I eat "right" most of the time, and *wrong* enough of the time to make eating fun. I take my breakfast malt three or four days a week and other mornings I eat bacon, eggs, buttered toast and I drink coffee with milk and two Sweet 'n Low packets; maybe two cups of coffee.

Sometimes I drink milk or orange juice instead.

I exercise a total of maybe 20 minutes every other day and I play golf three or four times a week—riding in a cart—and I drive as close as I am allowed to the ball to keep my golf etiquette intact. I am 5' 11¾" and weight about 183 pounds as a rule. When I started with Calorad I had "grown" to 191 pounds.

The second day on Calorad, I used a Body Fat Meter to measure my body fat. It showed 17.4% body fat. Within two weeks (still sleeping soundly each night and experiencing surprisingly other physical responses upon awakening that I can't specify), I lost 12 pounds in 14 days and my face became thinner and my stomach flatter. I lost an inch or two from my waist. I didn't measure prior to taking Calorad, I just *know* there's more room between my body and my pants at the waistline.

In the following two weeks I gained four pounds, but my appetite lessened; I now eat one full meal a day instead of two or three, and I'm never hungry. It's been three months now and the electronic Body Fat Meter showed 13% body fat! I'm told it isn't as accurate as the water weighing process. The fact is, I DON'T CARE! The same meter showed that my body fat went *down* more than 22% in 90 days. And, I **feel** terrific!

I had to travel for about ten days and didn't exercise. When I went back to my exercise machine to do sit up presses, I glanced back at the weights thinking my neighbor's teenage son had been using the machine and reduced the poundage. He hadn't! I added 20 pounds of weight and have been doing three sets of 25 but with an increase of about 20% in strength. I can only attribute that strength gain to my taking Calorad.

Without a doubt, the "good things" that have happened to me were after I began using Calorad. I have more energy, my body weight has been right at 181 pounds and the sinus headaches I experienced often over the past 15 years have completely disappeared.

After meeting with Michel Grisé at breakfast and having coffee with my meal, he asked that I use only *raw sugar:* "It assimilates better in the body and is healthier for you." I also began drinking more water.

Another Couple:

My buddy, a 39-year-old golf pro, is about 40 pounds overweight and had trouble with an arthritis-like pain. His name is Newton Pinkney Hartline (we call him Pinkey) and he is the Director of Golf at Freeport Golf Club in Freeport, Texas.

The first night he took Calorad and every night since, he slept soundly and felt rested in the morning. He lost 11 pounds in 14 days and inches from his blossoming waistline. He had to take six to eight anti-inflammatory pills EACH MORNING in order to eliminate this stiffness. Within six days, he no longer had pain and discontinued the medication.

It's been three months now that he has been using Calorad. He has lost a total of 26 pounds but he is eating *more!* His shoulder and neck pain has disappeared and he is playing more golf than ever before.

His wife, Carrie, is voluptuous (what you might call "stacked") and in the past 14 months since taking a job as a dental assistant, she gained 20 pounds. Within two weeks of being on Calorad, she lost several inches from her waist, hips and thighs and REALLY looks great again. She says her sleep is more restful and uninterrupted. She didn't weigh before she started and refuses to weigh now. She is happily losing inches.

It's now been three months on Calorad for her, too. She went from a LARGE to a SMALL size in *Llz Claiborne* dresses and pant suits. Her only complaint is the cost of buying new (smaller) clothes and having to alter the ones she had been wearing. She is absolutely thrilled over this weight and inch loss and so is her husband, Pinkey.

Another friend:

Rudy Hebert is in his early fifties. About 30 years ago, Rudy was the 13th strongest man in the world in his weight class of 160 pounds. He now weighs about 200, and works out three days a week with weights but not on body building, just sessions to see how much he can still bench press, curl, jerk, etc. He was a total nonbelieiver.

"I'll try your *stuff* Pedro," he told me after about three weeks of my badgering him. "But you know I don't believe in it."

Within two weeks Rudy's bench press went up 25 pounds, and he is thrilled. "My legs don't hurt any more and my torn shoulder feels better, I swear! I've lost a few inches from my waist and I feel better."

This, I realize, is not something to make any of you run out and buy a bottle of Calorad, but it really *is* something huge, if you knew Rudy. And 25 pounds when you are already bench pressing 300 is really awesome. When you press heavy weights, two or three pounds is a large increase. But to have 25 all of a sudden "happen" is breath-taking to a lifter. He's had that increase in strength for about three weeks now.

I didn't tell any of these folks anything but what Calorad had done for me, and the Calorad people only give out testimonials written to them by Calorad users. I scanned all of their brochures and written material and saw no place where they make a fat loss or weight loss claim, only personal testimonies by users.

I know they are under rules by the FDA but this doesn't apply to those rules because Calorad is not a drug, it is not a synthetic, it contains no stimulants; it is an ALL NATURAL food! It harms no one and can only help. I believe in it so strongly because it has made only positive changes in my life, and on the lives of friends and relatives. Since beginning work on this book, I have given out Calorad to over 90 people and received positive results on all but three individuals.

One used it for two weeks and quit. The other needs to lose maybe 40 pounds, eats as if he's going to be electrocuted after his last meal, follows the three-hour-no-eating before sleep plan but "manages" to devour a bowl of ice cream before bed which he doesn't count. The third one was my friend from my golf club who just said it didn't work on him.

TESTIMONIALS

☆ LOST WEIGHT
☆ LOST INCHES
☆ INCREASED ENERGY
☆ SLEPT SOUNDLY
☆ AGE SPOTS RECEDED

ENTIRE FAMILY BENEFITS . . . .

"I hold a Doctorate in clinical nutrition, specialize in preventive nutrition, and am involved in Post Doctoral Research in nutrition at Ohio State University. I wanted to fully research Calorad through Medline and the Internet before I recommended it to friends and acquaintances, so I didn't begin immediately.

"As a scientist and full time Cardiovascular Research Consultant and Oncology Disease Specialist working for a major pharmaceutical company, I am prohibited by company policy from discussing any 'part-time' business venture during normal working hours. In addition to this restriction, I spend a great deal of time out-of-state as part of my job requirements.

"I am an officer in the Marine Corps Reserve, I serve as Executive Director to The Ohio Chapter of the American College of Preventive Nutrition, and am an active member of the Executive Board of Directors of the Franklin County Chapter of the American Heart Association (AHA), and volunteer for AHA committee.

"I personally have lost almost 12 pounds and over 2½ inches off my waist within my first four weeks on Calorad and my wife Lynn lost three pounds and a total of five inches at the same time. I have increased energy, improved sleep, and have also seen several *lipofuscin deposits* (age spots) on my hands recede and totally disappear.

"My wife previously suffered from frequent and rather severe bouts of insomnia, but now "sleeps like a baby." My teenage son and daughter also use the product and have seen weight loss and muscle toning as a result of their Calorad use. My sister lost 10 pounds and two dress sizes in three weeks and loves the product."

Steven P. Perrosino, Ph.D., FACPN
Dublin, Ohio

PATIENTS LOST WEIGHT, INCREASED ENERGY . . .

"My Ph.D. is in clinical nutrition and I've been working in the nutritional field for 16 years. One of my focus areas is tracking people's health problems to their root as nutritional deficiencies. From my broad experience researching health in relation to nutrition, I recognize Calorad as a product that is positively needed by everyone, whether they have a weight problem or not.

"My experience with this product has been astounding. My patients, under less than ideal stress conditions, are losing weight and inches and gaining energy. Calorad stimulates a source of natural energy in the body and those who are taking it are becoming self-evident testimonials to the power of this incredible wellness resource. There is no need to "try out" this product. It is an important source of nutrition for all bodies alike and it works. I would say it's the next universal juice drink."

Dr. Robert Fahey, Ph.D.
Honolulu, HI

LOST 14 POUNDS IN THREE WEEKS . . . .

"I am a Registered Nurse/Hospital Admini-strator and my husband, a chiropractor. I started taking Calorad on March 8, 1997. I was initially skeptical about how this worked, but have always said 'when they find something that will let me lose weight while I sleep that I would try it.' I did, and it worked. My husband is 6' 2" and lost 14 pounds in three weeks, from 187 to 173. I have lost eight pounds and 15 inches in four weeks and am still losing, but more slowly now. I am very happy we found Calorad."

Kay White, MSN, RN
San Marcos, TX

20 PATIENTS LOSE WEIGHT and INCHES . . . .

"I have been looking for a collagen-based product like Calorad for over 20 years. I have repeatedly asked manufacturers to formulate a product like Calorad to no avail. When I saw Calorad's ingredient set, I got in touch with a principal from the company. I checked the product out thoroughly and put 20 patients on the product.

The success rate was incredible. I love this product for a number of important reasons. "Firstly, this is a totally unique product. I know this because, besides my large professional practice, I have owned and operated four health food stores in the last 27 years. There is nothing on the market like Calorad. I like the delivery system. It is simple and elegant. Without changing any major behaviors, my patients are losing weight and more importantly, inches.

"Beyond the weight management success, I believe that Calorad supports people that are experiencing nutritional deficiencies. This is an important product for people who live in large cities and experience the toxicity endemic to urban populations.

"I have built a very large and extensive group of health practitioners and lay distributors. All this because I believe in the product and everyone sees the merit of the product almost immediately. My customers and my colleagues say *'yes'* to Calorad. I am pleased and amazed while doing well."

Dr. Ed Wagner, D.C.
Malibu, CA

Evelyn Franks, poster girl of New Jersey

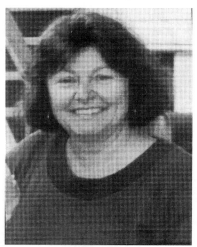

Before

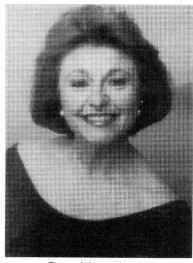

One Year Later

CALORAD's POSTER GIRL OF NEW JERSEY. . . . .

"I had a weight problem but also a multitude of other ailments. I was catching cold after cold. Congestion made breathing difficult. I had allergy flare-ups, sinusitis, headaches, bloating, gas, heel spurs and weak nails. My triglycerides were up to 1,490 and cholesterol of 325. I had pre menopausal problems, hot flashes and night sweats. My bladder felt as if it wouldn't hold water anymore. At 53, I was a wreck! Janice Picking, my nutritionist, put me on Calorad and Agrisept-L.

"It's been a year now. I've dropped 40 pounds and numerous inches. My body looks as if has been re-sculpted. I have rid myself of all the conditions that were aggravating me. My triglycerides are now 125 and my cholesterol dropped 100 points. I no longer need to take menopausal medication. I lost my double chin and the skin around my eyes has tightened. My upper arms have trimmed down and the cellulite behind my thighs is GONE! I sleep better and can handle stress. I have a brand new life!"

Evelyn Franks
Cape May, New Jersey

86% WHO TRY CALORAD REPORT BENEFITS . . . . . .

"As a licensed nutritionist and health food store owner with 30 years experience in the health and nutrition field, I feel confident that Calorad is truly a unique and health-promoting product. Approximately 86% of our customers who try Calorad are reporting benefits! I am also impressed with other nutritional support products in EYI's line and like the way they dovetail together in supporting the total health of the individual.

"My staff and I have shared Calorad with others in the health care field and now have chiropractors, massage therapists, acupuncturists and others all distributing the product."

George Miller
Naples, FL

ENERGY, STAMINA & MUSCLE TONE FROM CALORAD

"My results with Calorad have been phenomenal! Personally, I take it during the day for energy and stamina. I don't need to lose any weight, but there's no denying the toning that's taking place in my body. My calves are harder and more defined, and my thighs are tighter. It's really quite remark-able.

"I've given Calorad to my patients with tremendous success. One woman took off seven lbs. in four days and is feeling noticeably more healthy and vibrant. A physician colleague of mine is seeing his abdomen muscles like never before and taking off pant sizes.

"A woman patient of mine who is generally in so much physical pain and has such low energy that she spends her days in bed, has informed me that she's been walking her dog and cleaning the house because she is so vitalized on Calorad. The ingredients in this product are completely safe and effective. There are no side effects. No bloating. No gas."

Dr. C. I. Middleton
Los Angeles, CA

LOSE WEIGHT WHILE YOU SLEEP BUILD LEAN MUSCLE

"I have been in the field of preventive health-care for over 20 years. I am dedicated to exposing people to the best options available to protect their health, and prevent disease. Because this is the main focus of my practice, I spend a lot of time *swimming upstream*. I am constantly trying to talk my patients into doing things that will improve their health (i.e., nutrition, exercise, lifestyle changes).

"I am thrilled to be able to make Calorad available to my patients! It is wonderful to recommend a product that is so healthy, and have all of my patients respond so excitedly! For the first time, I don't feel like I'm swimming upstream. Everyone seems to want the benefits of lean muscle, and tissue regeneration, and of course, many people would like to take off a few pounds in their sleep! This product is fantastic!

Dr. Kerry L. Diliberg
Kauai, Hawaii

PERSONAL TRAINER TO WIN CHAMPIONSHIPS . . . . .

I thought you might be interested in a day in the life of Greg Sumner: Personal Trainer, Nutritional Consultant, National Power Lifting Champion with four world records, and Silver Medalist in the Masters World Championships. Here's the scoop on his first week of results with Calorad:

". . . My first client of the day was Cheri Lerma who just won the State Power Lifting Championships, setting four state records. She seemed rather strong this particular morning. I passed it off figuring she might have had a few good meals and lots of rest. It was nothing compared to what my next client accomplished in her workout.

"We were doing a leg workout the previous week and it was a major ordeal to get the Power Lifting Belt to the first notch. I almost gave up but we finally combined our strength and did it.

"One week later she comes in weighing five pounds less and pulled the belt to the second notch all by herself and squatted 40 pounds more weight! I know she could have done more too! I was and am very impressed.

Greg Sumner
Seaside, OR

LOST 22 POUNDS IN 11 WEEKS and CHRONIC PAINS RELIEVED . . . .

"I've been a chiropractor for 20 years and have owned multiple chiropractic clinics. I was a pharmaceutical representative for over five years

prior to becoming a chiropractor. I have not en-
countered a weight management product that
comes even *close* to the effectiveness and won-
derful results that are obtained with Calorad.
Personally, I lost 22 pounds in my first 11 weeks
on Calorad. I purposely ate all the foods I enjoyed
and avoided exercise in order to prove the product.
Boy, did it work!

"I lost four notches in my belt, my chronic
bilateral knee pain of 28 years and chronic right
shoulder pain of 21 years have been resolved. My
patients are getting very similar and wonderful
results. I recommend every Chiropractor in the
world to use Calorad personally and profession-
ally."

Bill Uriarte, D.C.
Windsor, CA

BODY BUILDER'S 3 P.M. ENERGY DIP GONE . . . .

"I am an avid body builder and have been
paying attention to personal fitness as a passion
for many years. I work out consistently, at least
four times a week and am acutely aware of the
way my body looks and feels. Since I've been

taking Calorad, I've noticed some tremendous changes in my physical well-being. For one, my energy level has evened out.

"My three o'clock dip has disappeared and I feel consistently healthy and energized. As far as my external appearance goes, I'm seeing definition and toning that is new and extremely exciting for me. In the last few weeks I've been inundated with people from the gym and elsewhere asking me what I'm doing that's working so well! I'm very happy and more fit than ever. "

Bob Scullion
Los Angeles, CA

AEROBICS INSTRUCTOR TRANSFORMS WITHOUT EXERCISE . . . .

"I am an aerobics instructor by trade. I didn't have any weight to lose coming into my Calorad experience and was curious to see what this "muscle-builder" would do for my body. Well, in my second month of taking the product I'm noticing some pretty incredible things. I do a lot of cardio-vascular exercise but have not been lifting at all since I started Calorad.

"Amazingly, my arms are now more defined than they were when I was lifting weights. I'm starting to see cuts in my leg muscles that have never come to the surface before. Just the other day I visited my massage therapist who has supported me as an athlete for ten years. He could not believe the enormous change in my body's muscle composition.

"He was blown away that the body he had been working on for 10 years had transformed so magnificently in just over a month. He wanted to know what I was doing and bought two bottles of Calorad immediately. I didn't know that I could feel better and stronger than I did a month ago, but Calorad has changed my life in some pretty significant ways."

Karla Yates
San Fernando, CA

FITNESS TRAINER LOSES INCHES FROM WAIST . . . .

"I am the owner and operator of *Executive Mobile Fitness.* My gift in life has been to train personally as well as to educate properly all facets of exercise, personalized fitness training programs, and health & wellness. I have been taking Calorad for four months and am experiencing increased cardiovascular fitness and substantial increases in the weight I lift. I have lost nine pounds of body fat, gained nine pounds of muscle back (per my body composition machine) and lost three and one-half inches off my waist line.

"My most dramatic physical changes have been three inches of muscle growth on my chest and back. Calorad is a tremendous product! I recommend it to my clients and everyone I meet!"

Michael Paul, N.A.S.M.C.P.T.
Lancaster, CA

DESIGNER GETS AMAZING RESULTS WITH CALORAD

"I started taking Calorad around the end of last September when a client of mine, Cheryl Ward, brought it to my attention. While I was on my first bottle people saw that I was losing weight. I didn't see it, but they did. Toward the end of my second bottle, I realized I was actually shrinking before my own eyes. By the end of the third bottle I had lost four inches off my waist, four inches off my hips. I was a totally transformed woman. I looked like a new person. I've been a designer for 20 years.

"My clients, who hadn't seen me in a while, started asking what was going on. In designing clothes for celebrities it was just a natural to help them find a way to look better in the clothes I designed for them. Before I looked up I had sold 20 bottles. My husband, Jonathan and I are building a terrific business with lots of wonderful friends. What a blessing this product is in our lives."

Angela Dean
Clothing Designer
Los Angeles, CA

EX-DIETER LOSES 40 INCHES IN FOUR WEEKS . . . . .

"I've done every diet that comes along, rice diets, high protein diets, straight vegetable diets, you name it, I tried it. I started taking Calorad and as of four weeks now, I have lost 15 lbs. and 40 inches all over my body, five inches in my abdomen, and five inches in my waist! I drink 80 ounces of water a day, approximately 2½ quarts, which I believe, along with the Calorad, is the winning combination. My cholesterol has gone down from

330 to 150 and instead of taking an average of 200 pain relievers a month for my arthritis. This month I only took six. I was going into X-large sizes. Now I can fit into size 14. I think Calorad is the greatest thing going!"

Judy Andrejski
Bay City, Michigan

SIZE TWENTY TO SIZE TEN . . . .

"I have had phenomenal results with the Calorad. When I started taking it, I was wearing a size 20. While on my second bottle, I went to the store to buy a new pair of jeans and discovered I could fit into a size 16! I lost 50 pounds in my first four months and went from a size 20 to a size 12. The next four months I lost an additional 16 pounds and continued losing inches. Today, I have lost a total of 64 pounds and am sporting a size 10 wardrobe, looking and feeling fabulous!"

Linda Jones
Spokane, Washington

POLICE CAPTAIN LOSES 90 POUNDS . . . .

"I am a Captain in the CRIM CT DIV responsible for the safety of 4,000 people each day. I am a 20-year veteran of the (New York Police) Force. I have personally lost 90 lbs. to date with the help of Calorad. I take it twice a day, every day, and I am convinced Calorad really works. I speak to anyone and everyone who will listen to me about the product."

Paul J. Christopher
Police Capt.
Merrick, NY

LOST 10 POUNDS AND RAISED HER TUSH . . . .

"I was planning on having to spend the rest of my life looking like a fat little Jewish grandmother. It's certainly not what I dreamed of for myself and the vision, quite frankly, made me very sad. Three weeks ago I started on Calorad, pretty desperate for something to work out for me. Within a matter of three days I could feel a shift taking place. In three weeks I've taken off 10 pounds without changing a thing in my life. My legs don't rub together, my arms don't pudge out, my stomach has gone down two inches and my tush has raised up. I never thought this could happen to me. It is beyond a dream come true."

Ava Gudeman
Los Angeles, CA

MARINE HAS BEST ABS EVER AFTER TWO WEEKS . . .

"I'm a massage therapist and a former Marine Corp. physical fitness instructor. I used to do weighted sit-ups with 50 lbs. behind my neck. You could kick me in the stomach and it wouldn't hurt me, but you couldn't see abs. After two weeks on Calorad I had better abs than I've had my whole life! My abs are cut! It's been 10 weeks now and I've gone from 173 to 160 on the scales and lost two inches in my waist. I'm training less, yet my leg muscles are more defined and I'm looking better than I have in a long time!"

Scott Stafford
Lewisberry, PA

FROM A TIGHT SIZE 22 to SIZE 16 IN JUST FIVE WEEKS

"In five weeks I've gone from a tight size 22 (had to push my belly in to zip up my jump suit jacket) to a snug 16! I've lost 11 pounds and 39½ inches. I've lost 18% of my body fat! Last week I gained a pound and lost 4½ inches and 4% body fat! If I wasn't measuring, I would have been discouraged with that one pound weight gain! I'm going through my closet, wearing clothes I haven't worn in years! Throwing out all my size 20's and 22's!

"And I weigh twenty pounds more than when I wore a size 16. I'm tightening! The best thing is the difference in how I think about myself! My friend commented that she notices a difference when she sees me at a distance; that I walk differently and carry myself differently. And I know why. I feel so good about myself. I am proud of myself. I am a real person again! And I love Sunday's. It's the day I weigh in and measure and Sunday has become my favorite day of the week."

Maria Iannuzzi
Wilkes-Barre, PA

RELIEF FROM RHEUMATOID ARTHRITIS WITH CALORAD

"I have had rheumatoid arthritis for several years. I had to quit working and go on disability because my disease got so bad. I couldn't get dressed to go to work in the morning because of stiffness and swelling. My fingers were so swollen I haven't been able to drive a car. The disease got me down. I've been on lots of pain medications, anti-inflammatories, and antidepressants. I have been basically house-ridden since October of '96.

"I started taking Calorad four weeks ago, and the swelling has gone down in my hands and my fingers look straighter. The pain is leaving the joints in my ankles and legs and I can walk without assistance. I can now drive and I just started going to the supermarket by myself again. I even took my dog to be groomed the other day. I have had so many good days since being on Calorad. I feel so much better. I'm regaining my independence again which is such a thrill!"

Eileen Malloy
Chambersburg, PA

BUFFY'S WEARING A DRESS THAT HASN'T FIT IN TEN
YEARS . . . .

"I have been battling weight all my life and losing the battle. I started on Calorad on November 26, 1996. I went to Florida over Christmas and New Years and put it to the test. This was the first time in 17 years that I didn't gain weight during the winter months. Since starting Calorad I have lost 24 lbs. and 20 inches. I started out in a size 20 and now I'm a size 16. I don't have to shop in the "plus size" stores anymore!

"I am the mother of four and I feel like I'm 20 again. I am going strong till midnight. The *carpel tunnel syndrome* I've had for 15 years is gone. I sleep soundly and wake up refreshed. I wore a dress to church that I haven't been able to fit into for 10 years. I got so many compliments. It was a wonderful feeling! I feel like I have control over where I am going for the first time in my life!"

Buffy Kasinec
Elyria, Ohio

FIGURE RESHAPED IN 30 DAYS . . . .

In June of 1996, I began taking Calorad to lose five to ten pounds. I experienced a two to three pound weight loss in the first 30 days, and I noticed my skin starting to improve, and a general feeling of well-being.

In the following month, my clothes began getting looser in the waist, hips and thighs as I had lost about two and a half inches overall. My total weight loss is about seven pounds now and one size smaller in my clothes.

I'm thrilled with this and continue to see a muscle tightening and reshaping of my figure. I am now within my ideal weight range and will continue taking Calorad for the rejuvenation I see and feel week by week.

Sabrina Dancy
Lake City, FL

LOST 15 POUNDS IN SIX TO SEVEN WEEKS . . . . . .

"I opened a retail store and have been operating it for four years now. I sell herbs, vitamins, homeopathic products, teas, books, and specialize in wellness and cleansing. Many people were coming in and asking, "What do you have for weight loss?" So, I bought five bottles of Calorad, used one on myself and lost 15 lbs. in six weeks.

"When Calorad began working for me, I decided to write an article for the Health and Fitness page of our local paper. People started calling the newspaper to find out about Calorad because they didn't know how to reach me. I had to pick up 36 bottles, 18 of which went out of the store in one day and I had people on a waiting list. I then had to close the store and put up a sign, 'Sorry, had to go to Santa Monica to pick up Calorad!'

"But that was only the beginning! The results have continued to fire up the demand. Today, I have a sign on the street outside my store that reads, *Lose Weight While You're Sleeping.* That draws people in and I give them a brochure and talk with them about Calorad. I can never stock enough Calorad."

Cathy Richer
Health Food Store Owner
Fallbrook, CA

HEALTH FOOD STORE MANAGER LOST 10 LBS. IN THREE WEEKS . . . .

"I currently manage a health food store that began offering Calorad to our retail customers three weeks ago. Already we have sold 140 bottles with 25 people on a waiting list for the next shipment! I've been in the health field for 25 years and watched products come and go. I really like Calorad because it contains no stimulants, no suppressants, has no side effects, and everybody can use it. In fact, I am impressed with the other products in the EYI line as well. Grapefruit Seed Extract has always worked well but it seems that the added citrus extracts in Agrisept-L may make it an even better formula.

"I have personally been on the product for three weeks now and have lost 10 pounds and 1½ inches around my waist. I also lost my craving for sweets. I feel so good and have so much energy that I went out and joined a gym. I am very pleased with Calorad to say the least!"

Jim Wilk
Health Food Store Manager
Lansdale, PA

*HAIRDRESSER HAS UNKNOWN AILS CURED ON THE
FIRST NIGHT'S USE OF CALORAD* . . . .

"For the past 12 years I have owned and operated *'For Ladies Only Beauty Salon.'* I heard about Calorad from a friend, Sue Hale, and it sounded wonderful. I planned to buy one bottle to see if it worked but it was so exciting listening about Calorad I decided to buy five bottles and try the business. I still didn't know exactly what I was going to do. I simply put a sign on the door that read: *Lose weight, no diet or exercise required.* And, I put some Calorad brochures on the counter. What a surprise!

"The very next day I had to call Ray in Los Angeles for five more bottles and by that night I had to call for five more. At first my customers wanted to wait to see what results I was going to have, but before I had been on Calorad even three days, they came back and said, 'Just give me a bottle now. You're going to be skinny and I'm not and then I'm going to be upset.'

"Also, I had been ill for the last year and on a lot of antibiotics. My energy was gone and I was just dragging. I was going to doctors and getting blood tests to try and find out what the problem was. After taking Calorad the first night, I couldn't believe it. I felt like my old self! My family and friends noticed the change right away and asked if I was OK. And then I sold it to all my friends because they saw my energy change."

Diane Napier
Beauty Salon Owner
Long Beach, CA

NON-BELIEVER LOSES 33½ INCHES and GETS PAIN UNDER CONTROL . . . .

Mid-September, 1996, my husband, Larry, gave me a brochure on Calorad. I admit, my reaction was not favorable. I took one look at "take one tablespoon of this clear liquid on an empty stomach with a glass of water just prior to sleep and wake up thinner," and in the trash it went. My husband retrieved it and gave it back to me several days later with a message from a very dear friend saying the product did work. I still thought it was a joke but since I had tried almost every other "diet" known, I said I would try.

It took exactly two weeks to go from skeptic to believer. From the very first night, I slept better than I ever had. Before Calorad, I very seldom slept more than four hours nightly and the slightest disturbance would keep me awake the rest of the night. Now I am sleeping a normal eight hours and if anything wakes me, I can get up and go right back to sleep! At the end of the first two weeks. It was time to measure again. I argued it was a waste of time for I felt I had not lost anything. To my amazement, I had lost an overall of 8½ inches. In as little as five months, I lost a total of 33½ inches and have changed dress sized from 24W to 18W. I am still on the product and still in the process of losing and reshaping (size 16 and losing.)

But as wonderful as the inch loss is, it is nothing compared to the real benefit I have received. In 1985 I had TMJ (jaw joint) surgery. In 1990, the implant failed and had to be removed. After the second surgery, I was having more and more trouble with that joint and the only option the doctor could offer me was another surgery. I was resigned to having pain in my jaw for the rest of my life which felt like a constant toothache. I was taking entirely too many pain relievers every day and using magnets every night for relief. After four months of using Calorad, my daily medication was greatly reduced. Since July 1997, I've used pain relievers only twice a month.

The last checkup with the surgeon was great. From the measurements he took, the range of motion was the same, or better than when I went to him before the first surgery!

Elaine Barbery
Houston, TX

****

Has this been exciting? Even after reading all of this there are skeptics but please, maybe for the first time in your life, take a chance to lose fat, feel and look better and **actually *be* healthier.**

We didn't PAY these people to give their testimonials; they volunteered them. And Calorad has been around a long time and is here to stay. It's worked wonders on so very many people and made their lives so very much better. Try it on yourself, please!

Also, remember that LOSING FAT is a *side effect* from using Calorad. My personal experience, and from interviewing hundreds who are taking the product, is that your ENERGY LEVEL increases almost instantly. From this, you automatically become more active and it *does* make you aware of eating more of the "right" foods, drinking more water, and staying away from the constant eating of "bad" foods, thus helping the entire plan work.

I still interview people who are on the program and I am constantly amazed at the results. It makes my life more fulfilling because I am a part of letting others know about this wondrous miracle that takes away INCHES and FAT. And, when your body loses fat, it repairs many ills.

I have a few dozen golf buddies from 40 to 72 years old and within only weeks of being on Calorad, their bones no longer squeak and snap when they first get up each morning. The collagen in Calorad lubricates their joints the same as grease does for rusted automobile springs.

And ladies, woefully, it seems to work faster on men, but regardless of your gender, Calorad will do wonders for the way you *feel.* If you are one of the overFAT, be patient. Remember, it took you years to get this way so give Calorad time to work.

I must have a few THOUSAND testimonials that are sent to me and more often than not, when I hear the wonders it's performed on so many, tears of joy well in my eyes. I feel good about myself. Being involved with Calorad has helped me physically, mentally, spiritually and if I sell as many

Chapter 4

FREQUENTLY ASKED QUESTIONS

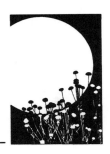

 What is Calorad?

 Calorad is a food as well as a weight management product. It's collagen formula supports the body in building lean muscle tissue. For those who carry around excess weight, the building of lean muscle tissue assists the body in utilizing sugars and fats more efficiently. For those who are trim and don't need to lose weight, Calorad supports the body in building strength and vitality.

 Is Calorad FDA approved?

 There is no need. It is a food supplement. No synthetics, no chemicals, no drugs, no stimulants; only protein, which is a food.

Q. Is it patented?

A. No! And that is a bright question. Michel Grisé neither needed nor wanted a patent. His formula is secret and others have tried to duplicate it but could not. Coca Cola is not patented either.

Q. I'm about 20 pounds overweight but my sister is trim. Should I take Calorad and forget about her?

A. Calorad is good for all body types. It is a *food supplement*, more specifically a *collagen* supplement, that enhances the body's natural mechanism of rejuvenation and repair. Everyone benefits from Calorad.

Q. Why does Calorad work?

A. These are medical facts: When we go to sleep at night, the first 45 to 90 minutes of sleep are a period of productivity in the body. Our minds go to rest, but our bodies go to work in a process of revitalization and repair. Calorad, when taken on a stomach empty of food for at least three hours with a glass of water directly before sleep, fuels and feeds that process. Just like any protein that builds the body, Calorad builds in a height-ened way when taken in this manner.

Q. Will I have to diet and begin (or increase) my exercise schedule?

A. **No and No!** The beauty of the program is that it is so simple. The cessation of food intake **three hours prior to sleep**, if not being done already, is the only stipulation, which in and of itself is a very healthy behavioral shift.

And, there's no need to diet. In most diets, 30% of your muscle mass is sacrificed for weight loss. With Calorad, the **building** of muscle is what incurs the weight reduction and, consequently, people lose inches as well as pounds. Remember, diet is *what* you eat, not *how much* you eat. So please eat healthy foods.

As far as exercise, do as little or as much as you were doing before Calorad. My personal experience, as well as from the testimonials in this text, is that the increased energy from taking Calorad should make you want to do more physi-cal activities

Q. How much weight will I lose?

A. That's hard to tell. Many people lose *inches* before they ever lose a pound, fitting differently in their clothes or perhaps dropping a dress/pant size without noticing any changes on the scale. Then, there are those who initially **put on** weight, but **lose inches** because muscle weighs **twice** as much as fat.

Q. How can I be assured that it will work on me and I'll lose fat?

A. **You can't!** You can only give it a trial. However, it works in positive ways of just about everyone judging from the testimonials. The results show up differently in each subjective body. Some will experience noticeable results in the first week and some not until the third month. Some will lose steadily at a very slow rate (for instance one pound every two weeks) and some will plateau out for a while and for others, fat just melts away. Remember, the **trial period** is 90 days! Trust me, it's worth the time.

Q. What else does Calorad do?

A. I can only tell you to go back through the many testimonials of what others claim happened to them once they began using Calorad.

In my interview with Michel Grisé, he pointed out to me how your skin becomes more elastic once it's sagged from age or weight. I talked with others who claim their age spots disappeared, of wrinkles vanishing, and even those who believed their hair grew.

At a meeting in Houston in September of 1997, one lady said she feared she would be totally bald, because her hair was falling out in clumps. "Within six weeks after beginning to use Calorad, it came back—but it was gray. I can dye it," she said. "I'm just so thrilled that its coming back regardless of the color."

I am not saying that Calorad will grow hair! In consulting with physicians, their explanation was that the lady apparently had a medical problem that her body corrected once the excess body fat was gone.

Q. Suppose it doesn't work on me at all?

A. For those 14% who do not experience any weight or fat loss, this could be due to latent thyroid problems, mineral deficiency, colon health, or personal chemistry. See a health practitioner to get these problems resolved, and *then* give Calorad a 90-day trial. It could change your life!

You will *still* benefit from the ingredients in Calorad much in the same way you benefit from taking vitamin or mineral supplements. There is **no** *wrong* **experience** from the product. It is simply life supporting in various ways for different people.

Q. How do I take Calorad for *optimum* weight management results?

A. As mentioned several times earlier in this book, one tablespoonful of Calorad should be taken directly before sleep, at least three hours after your last meal, with a full, eight ounce glass of water. You can mix it with water or drink them separately. I like to mix it in **cold** water and I keep my Calorad in my refrigerator. No reason. I just like it cold.

Now remember, it is also healthier to **drink 8 to 10 glasses of water each day** to help cleanse your system. Along with that, adopt smart eating habits, and avoid the fat-causing foods as much as possible.

Remember, if you plan to read or watch television, you should **wait** to drink Calorad until you **finish** those activities. Calorad works best if the stomach is empty of food for at least three hours and you should take it just as your head hits the pillow. The plan *still works* if you eat during those three hours prior to sleep, but it works **better** if you follow that three-hour-no-eat or drink rule.

Q. How do I take Calorad for energy and stamina?

A. Calorad works to sustain daytime energy levels when taken in the above "nighttime" manner. But, for endurance and stamina, Calorad can also be taken during the day approximately **one half hour** before meals. Athletes can take Calorad 30 to 45 minutes before working out to support endurance and strength.

One friend of mine, a power lifter named Rudy Hebert, whom I mentioned earlier (who had to be convinced to take Calorad—no, I *badgered*

him, remember, but only because I care) is shout-
ing Calorad's praises all over Texas and Louisiana
because he has been bench pressing about 8%
more after being on Calorad only two weeks.

He said he had been stuck on a certain
weight for over five years prior to this. And, 8% is
a *lot* when you get up into the hundreds of pounds.

Q. How should I take Calorad if I don't want to
take off weight?

A. Calorad is, primarily, a *nutritional supple-
ment.* Individuals who need to lose excess
pounds and inches experience these results with
Calorad because it supports the body in building
muscle mass and, consequently utilizes fats and
sugars *more efficiently.* Calorad is not exclusively
for any one body type, however. It can be taken by
all physical types alike as a strength optimizer and
nutritional support product. For individuals taking
Calorad as a nutritional supplement, either of the
above methods are appropriate for usage.

Q. Can I take Calorad if I'm taking other vita-
mins and minerals? How about if I'm on
medication?

A. **Yes and Yes!** Calorad works with virtually *all* other nutritional supplements; that's the great part. However, it is suggested that if you take other nutritional supplements, take them with your **last meal** to maximize the efficacy of Calorad. Calorad works best when there is no other activity in the digestive system. Remember, drink water, water, water.

Similarly, if you have any questions about the compatibility of your medication with Calorad, it is suggested you take a bottle of Calorad with you to a health practitioner before proceeding.

Q. What if I don't lose any weight the first 30 days on Calorad?

A. That happened with three of the people I sold a single bottle of Calorad to. One friend at Hillcrest Golf Club, Joe DeJongh, took a bottle to lose weight. I had been using Calorad for two weeks when I mentioned it to him. I had lost 12 pounds so I was a believer.

I called Joe about 25 days after he began taking Calorad to find out what he had lost. "The price I paid for that stuff," Joe replied, laughing. "But I sleep better and I feel better." The **true test** is **90** days.

Q. NOW for the BIG QUESTIONS. WHERE do I get Calorad and is it expensive?

A. Calorad is not sold in ANY large retail stores; it is sold mostly through independent distributors and small business owners. Chances are it can be purchased in the very city in which you live. And, the price is less than a dinner for two at a nice restaurant and varies between countries. I'll tell you precisely where you can get it at the end of this book.

****

With Calorad and Agrisept-L, I literally **shove** it on those I love and care for. At first, I gave it to them but when they didn't use it, I jerked it back and made them pay.

On others, I simply *expose* them to it and if they read my book, they buy Calorad. I take the book with me wherever I go and when people see it, they automatically pick it up to read.

I must have done some wonderful thing in my life to have found Calorad. God does watch over each of us. When He guided the EYI group together to bring Calorad to Houston to find me and then enable me to write this book that could bring healthier lives to countless thousands, I know

I've been blessed. What a wonderful life I now have. And you, dear readers, have a happy, healthy wonderful life too. May God bless you all.

Pete Billac

DISCLAIMER

As the author, I mention several times in this book that I am not a physician nor a health professional of any kind; I am simply a writer who came across an amazing product that I want to share with mankind.

The information in this text is from my active and extensive research in soliciting the aid of physicians, nutritionist, chiropractors, pharmacists, and health practitioners, and from interviews with the brilliant man who formulated Calorad. From the Internet, I was able to get the testimonials I've chosen to include.

None of these people, in any form or fashion, are to be held responsible for whatever I've written in this book. Without their help I would have had little to say and I interpreted what they told me and what has been written about Calorad to the best of my ability.

Chapter 5

CALORAD FOR PETS

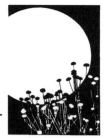

"Products that sound too good to be true usually are. Calorad is an exception. It is the only product I have actively endorsed during my 28 years as a veterinarian I have seen with my own eyes what this amazing nutrient can do. It is, without question, much more than a safe and effective weight loss product—it is a total body wellness supplement!

"I now have approximately 500 dogs, cats, and birds on Calorad as well as over 500 pet owners and friends. It is a great source of satisfaction for me to hear from people every single day that they are benefitting from the product or that their pets are. Animals become rejuvenated, i.e. dogs start acting like puppies after being on Calorad one day to three weeks.

"I have found Calorad supplement to be very useful in treating the older pet who is slowing down, sleeping a lot, and doesn't have as much enthusiasm. However, I also recommend the Calorad supplement for the middle aged, healthy, active pets to maintain a healthy situation for as long as possible, staying playful, active and out of pain.

"Pets have a shorter life span than humans and I believe Calorad can help to postpone the inevitable deterioration of these pets as long as possible.

A Golden Treat supplement (with Calorad in it) can improve many health situations including:

✔ to counteract the signs of aging
✔ to increase coat luster
✔ to aid in weight reduction
✔ for pets with slipped disks
✔ to improve energy levels
✔ for any pet exhibiting slow healing
✔ to help pet rebuild while recovering from serious medical or surgical illnesses and injuries
✔ to maintain youthful qualities such as playfulness
✔ to improve mobility and slow down joint degeneration in arthritic pets
✔ to help slow down or reverse muscle atrophy and weakness
✔ for pets with fatty livers or elevated blood fat levels
✔ to help lower blood sugars in diabetic pets
✔ for hypothyroid pets along with thyroid supplementation
✔ to help reduce fatty tumors in pets
✔ to minimize the side effects of long term cortisone therapy which can result in fatty liver, weak muscles and thin skin
✔ for the normal healthy pet, to help maintain wellness

Prevention is better than cure!

Chuck Galvin, D.V.M.
Novato, CA

ABOUT DR. CHUCK GALVIN

Dr. Galvin is a world renowned veterinarian with an extremely popular clinic that has attracted much media attention.

He was an original charter member of the Association of Avian Veterinarians—one of the fastest growth veterinary organizations in the world having thousands of members.

Dr. Galvin has been an international lecturer on pet bird care and published articles in journals and books. He is also a new friend.

ACKNOWLEDGMENTS

There is a long list of people to thank for the production of this book and I'll do my best to mention them all. I am so very, very grateful. Many of you I've never met.

My initial thanks goes to my friend, Dr. Carl Bechtel, who introduced me to this amazing product that has made my life and the lives of many close to me both healthier and happier. Next, I thank Jay Sargeant, The Director of U.S. Operations for Essentially Yours Industries, for a truly passionate speech he gave in Houston that motivated me to the point that I couldn't sleep for days thinking of those I loved and cared for that I could help—IF "this stuff" worked—and it has. Jay is a good person, warm, caring, and truly sincere.

I thank Geraldine Heyman, Director of International Sales and Marketing for Essentially Yours Industries, who had an idea and a plan and built a team of talented and caring people just like herself. She is a wonderful person, a sweetheart with boundless energy. I'd also like to thank her Fax machine; Geraldine is constantly traveling, but her Fax machine resides at the home office in Vancouver and enables me to "talk" to her.

And to Michel Grisé, the brilliant formulator who introduced several of the products that have enriched the quality of life for countless people. He is warm, human, caring and dedicated to helping others. He formulated Calorad and Agrisept-L, both trademarked. His amazing discoveries have been a major benefit to so very many. The exact number is difficult to determine but from an educated guess, maybe as many as a million people or more across the globe.

And, to Jerry Schoonover, a hypnotist and college counselor, who is a Calorad user and distributor in Houston, Texas. Jerry sent me information that helped enormously. I can't neglect to mention Ruby Miller-Lyman; I heard her speak on Calorad, too, and what I learned from Jay, she seconded in her up-beat, flowing style. She's a salesperson, *par excellence*, and I was amazed at her energy and vitality and her work habits. She travels the country speaking everywhere and her warmth and sincerity is simply awesome.

Then, a guy by the name of Jim Darechuk,

born in Canada now living in Houston, has been my mentor for understanding Calorad and the people involved. He is successful with his business because money is not his main motivating factor; it's helping others. And, of course, if you help enough people, money follows. I thank his partner, Priest Kemper and their associate, Ken Foley. The three men are truly terrific and they each helped me understand the importance this book might play on the health and happiness of others.

I met even more wonderful people at a large meeting in Jacksonville, Florida in November of 1997; the lovely Sabrina Dancy and her equally lovely sister, Audrey Taylor. They laughed at my 15-minute fun talk. How could I not like them? In thinking out loud, I've said to myself often. "What is it with these Essentially Yours people? How can they *all* be so doggoned sweet and caring and wonderful? Is it the energy they get from Calorad that gives them this attitude?"

There is little doubt, from my investigative research, that the majority of the over 275,000 Independent Distributors in this company are special. They became involved because Calorad worked on them and, like me, they wanted to share their "discovery" with others, especially those close to them. The money they can earn is secondary. I am convinced of that.

Now, for the company. Before I begin, know this: I have not been paid, coerced or prompted by anyone involved with Essentially Yours Industries.

What I'm going to share with you, like most of what I've written in the book, is what I read about, experienced and observed. I think the product, Calorad, has a magnetism about it. According to the February 1998 issue of MONEY MAKER'S MONTHLY, "EYI has created an awesome team of over 200,000 Independent Business Associates and is generating over *eight million dollars a month* in revenue. Many would say this would be an enviable record for a company which has been in existence for five to seven years—but EYI has been in business only two years!"

I agree that this phenomenal business success is due to the amazing discovery of Calorad, but it is also the "team" I spoke of that has been built from the top people in the company. A product alone, no matter how wondrous, isn't enough. And the team is expanding.

The likes of Al Pirnia, and Dr. John Norris, don't "just happen" to a company, they are *drawn* to us by a higher power the same as everyone finds Calorad.

If you missed the '98 convention in Orlando, you missed an experience. I have never in my entire life come away from any event so pumped, happy and proud to be associated with all of you, and I say that with utmost sincerity from my heart.

It simply all *must* go back to Geraldine Heyman, Michel and Louise Grisé, Jay Sargeant, Brian Lavorato (you have to love him instantly) and

Barry LaRose. I've now met them all. My new friends are Dave and Bonnie White, Linda Wright, Jean and Ted Vickers, Dr. Jerry Koch, and Dr. Mark Evans, and Dr. Luis Garg—all, very, very special; truly extraordinary people.

And to people like Rena Davis, Dr. Pamela Hiti, Ted and Joyce Brooks, Jack Herd, Art Burleigh, and my new telephone friends and editors, Stuart Purcell and Dr. Chuck Galvin. Where have all you wonderful people been hiding most of my life? Regardless, I welcome you.

From these parting remarks, it would appear that I am an officer or investor in the company. *I am neither.* I even resigned my distributorship because I do NOT sell Calorad; I write, publish and market books.

Calorad, as a product, has made a profound difference in my physical well being. I have more energy, more stamina, gotten rid of lots of nagging ills such as sinus headaches, being unable to sleep soundly, NO MORE SNORING, a heel spur that I had for over two years, my weight is down a permanent 10 pounds and my body fat went down over 22% in maybe 10 weeks. My chest is bigger, waist smaller, muscles tighter. It truly IS a miracle!

As a way to help others, it has changed my spiritual life. I feel good about what I'm doing. I like it. I love it. I embrace it.

LOSE FAT WHILE YOU SLEEP
is available through:

Swan Publishing
126 Live Oak
Alvin, TX 77511

(281) 388-2547
Fax (281) 585-3738

or e-mail: swanbooks@ghg.net

Visit our web page at:
www.swan-pub.com

To Order CALORAD
through an
Independent Distributor, Call

ABOUT THE AUTHOR

PETE BILLAC is one of the most sought-after speakers in the United States. He is billed as an Author/Lecturer/Humorist. Pete is a maverick; he writes only what pleases him. He has written 43 full-length books, hundreds of short stories and conducts fun lectures on cruise ships. His topics range from adventure and war, to famous people, history, self-help, health and romance.

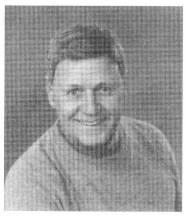

Perhaps you've seen him on Donahue, Sally Jessy Raphael, Good Morning America or any of the other network televison shows. He speaks to Fortune 500 companies on marketing, school kids on reading and writing, and to folks over 60 on keeping physically fit and enjoying life. He makes his audiences laugh . . . hard!

This book, LOSE FAT WHILE YOU SLEEP, is his favorite. His runaway best seller, HOW NOT TO BE LONELY, has sold over 4 million copies. "I feel this will do as well as Lonely," Pete says. "It will absolutely help everyone live a healthier and, hopefully, happier life."

Phil Donahue said, "Pete is an expert at restoring self-confidence and self-esteem in others."

Ken Collins, Syndicated Radio Celebrity Host said, "One of the funniest, most charismatic speakers I have ever heard. He breathes life into every topic. Be sure to attend any function where Pete is featured."